‒ GRIEF ‒
Survivor

28 STEPS TOWARD HOPE & HEALING

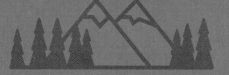

BETH MARSHALL

Beth Marshall
Grief Survivor
28 steps toward Hope and Healing

ISBN 978-0-9725903-4-1

Cover Design and Page Layout by Cody Bridenbaugh
Creative Consulting by Kathryn Helt

Editing by Heidi Charalambous and Meredith Higgins

WORDS OF APPRECIATION

Thanks to my friend and Senior Pastor of NewSpring Church, Perry Noble. Thousands of lives have been impacted by your transparent teaching that it's OK to not be OK. Thankfully, we don't have to stay that way.

Thanks to Cody Bridenbaugh, Kathryn Helt, Meredith Higgins, Sherry Cooley, Heidi Charalambous and Melissa Peacock for your creative contributions, encouragement and editing expertise.

Most of all, thanks to my husband, Paul for believing in me. Your unwavering love and support make my heart smile. I love you!

STEPS

INTRODUCTION

It's 10 o'clock at night and the phone rings. There is no warning—only the crushing news that someone you love is gone. You didn't even get to say goodbye. Or maybe you anticipated what was about to happen for weeks, months or even years. Whether the loss was sudden or there was time to prepare, the death of someone you care about can leave you with more questions than answers. Why didn't I get to say goodbye? How will I get through this?

After losing three close family members in five years, I remember feeling overwhelmed, as waves of unanticipated emotion would roll in like a storm. How long would this intense sorrow last? Would life ever feel normal again? What if I forget about them? And why do well-intentioned people say crazy things when they're trying to be helpful?

I searched volumes of grief-related books, envisioning a clear, concise manual to lead me down the well-lit path to healing. Surely there's a book to tell me exactly what to expect, how long this will take and when life will be back to normal. As you might imagine, there's no such book. Nothing on the market seemed to touch the deep grief in my heart. One morning, I finally found a comforting place to go with my pain. In the spiral notebook I used as a journal, I began to write through my grief.

You may be thinking right now: I'm not a writer. I don't like to write. Writing feels like school. Hold on. Please don't stop reading.

In Grief Survivor you'll find real-life tips for:
- knowing what you might expect,
- navigating holidays and other special days,
- taking care of yourself first so you'll be able to help others,
- knowing when to call for help,
- gaining confidence that your loved one will not be forgotten.

Whether you write on every page or simply read and reflect, I invite you to take the first step toward healing with Grief Survivor. ▪

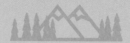

"Being kind to yourself is one of the wisest ways to help not only yourself but others who depend on you."

STEP 1

PUT ON YOUR OXYGEN MASK FIRST

You've probably heard it a million times. The flight crew reminds you to put your oxygen mask on before helping others. Grief survival is a lot like in-flight safety. Without oxygen, it's impossible help anyone else.

Regaining your equilibrium after loss can be physically and emotionally demanding. Taking good care of yourself is essential to staying strong enough to keep the other plates in your life spinning. Being kind to yourself is one of the wisest ways to help not only yourself but others who depend on you.

Rest is not a four-letter word. Technically it is, but not the bad kind. Rest is not laziness. Rest is OK, and rest doesn't have to mean doing nothing. Here are some examples of what that could look like.

- Turn off the noise of 24-hour news channels.
- Get to bed at a decent hour.
- Enjoy some fresh air, sunshine if possible, and a walk.
- Take a nap.
- Get a massage.
- Meet a friend for dinner.

Even if you don't have a cruise on the calendar this month, consider doing something kind for yourself every day.

What are 10 kind things you could do for yourself? Write them here, and do one today. ■

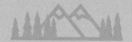

"Prayer, meditation, or listening to refreshing music are excellent ways to overcome fear and worry."

STEP 2

BE STILL

What's the first thing you do in the morning? Watch the news? Work out? Read the newspaper?

One of the best ways to find peace in the midst of a storm is to set aside a little time at the beginning of your day to be still. Before you check emails, drive carpools or race into your day, would you take a few moments to calm your mind?

Find a quiet place away from distractions. Reading from an inspirational book or devotional can help you overcome anxious thoughts and face the day with confidence. Prayer, meditation, or listening to refreshing music are excellent ways to overcome fear and worry.

How will you spend the first precious moments of your day tomorrow? Plan ahead. What will you listen to or read? Write your ideas on the following pages. ■

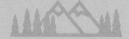

*"There's no formula for the
right way to grieve."*

STEP 3

YOU'RE THE BOSS

You're the only one who can determine how this season of grief will look. There's no formula for the right way to grieve. As long as you're not injuring yourself or anyone else, you're doing fine. As you take your first steps toward healing remember:

- When you feel like crying, cry.
- You may feel more relief than sadness right now. That's OK, too.
- If reminiscing and sharing stories about your loved one make you laugh, by all means do it.
- Steer clear of people and events that leave you anxious and exhausted. Choosing your activities and company wisely can prevent unnecessary stress.
- It's OK to say yes to the best, and no to the rest.
- White space on your calendar doesn't mean you're lazy.
- There's no need to apologize. You are the boss of your schedule.

Could changes in your schedule help minimize your stress? Use these pages for ideas on what changes you could make. ■

GRIEF SURVIVOR

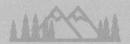

"Thankfully, most of the side effects grief causes—sleeplessness, appetite changes, an inability to stop crying—will lessen and eventually subside over time."

STEP 4

AM I DOING THIS RIGHT?

Have you ever walked into a room and turned around because you have no idea why you're there? Grief can do that to you. Unfamiliar emotions can make you think you're losing your mind and can make important decisions seem close to impossible. If you're experiencing mental fogginess you're not alone.

In the aftermath of loss, sleep may be a distant memory. You lay your head on the pillow, but your mind keeps racing with worries and anxious thoughts about tomorrow. Surely there's a way to get some sleep. The sun comes up, and you're not convinced you ever closed your eyes.

Mealtime may have been a time to refresh, laugh and share events of the day. Now the thought of food might seem unappealing. Or maybe you aren't able to eat enough, wondering if one more bite of luscious chocolate cake might help fill the hole in your heart.

Thankfully, most of the side effects grief causes—sleeplessness, appetite changes, an inability to stop crying—will lessen and eventually subside over time. The good news is you aren't going crazy.

Have you noticed changes in your appetite, mental clarity or sleep patterns? What has changed? How are you coping with those changes?

Make a list of how these parts of your life are different (if at all)— times when you struggle to make decisions, conversations and events that cause you to overeat or lose your appetite, thoughts that keep you up at night. ■

SURVIVAL TIP

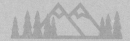

"What do you do when you can't sleep?"

STEP 5

I NEED SOME SLEEP!

What do you do when you can't sleep?

Here are a few ideas to help:
- Turn off cell phones, computers or tv an hour before bedtime.
- Cut out caffeine after 3 p.m.
- Listen to soothing music instead of late night news.
- Drink some caffeine-free, "sleepy-time" tea.
- Pray for peaceful rest.

Comforting words from Matthew 11:28: "Come to me all who are weary and burdened, and I will give you rest."

What changes could you make tonight to help you get some peaceful sleep? ■

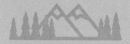

"...two or three weeks down the road the last casserole dish has been washed, flowers are faded and everyone seems to have vanished."

STEP 6

WHERE DID EVERYBODY GO?

The days immediately following a death are often overflowing with decisions, houseguests, flowers and meals being delivered. All the activity can serve as a welcome distraction from the reality of what has happened.

But two or three weeks down the road the last casserole dish has been washed, flowers are faded and everyone seems to have vanished. Countless people said, "Call if you need anything," but there was nothing you really needed. Now it would be nice for the phone to ring or for someone to stop by.

It might not feel comfortable at first, but would you consider letting someone know you're feeling lonely? You may want to ask a neighbor or friend to go for a walk or stop by for coffee. Most people are happy to help if they know there's a need.

If you're feeling isolated today, consider changing your routine. If you feel up to meeting someone for lunch or going to see a movie, call a friend.

What is one step you could take today to let someone know you would appreciate a little company? ▪

SURVIVAL TIP

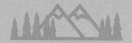

"Your lifelines through sorrow are often people who have walked a path similar to what you're going through."

STEP 7

LIFELINES

A trusted friend can be the lifeline that keeps you afloat. Maybe the people you thought would stay close are nowhere to be found; but someone you wouldn't have expected is right there by your side. Your lifelines through sorrow are often people who have walked a path similar to what you're going through.

In *Overwhelmed*, pastor Perry Noble puts it this way: *"...whatever is tearing you up inside, stop hiding it. The sooner you ask for help and admit you need other people, the sooner you will find relief."* [1]

Is there someone you can call anytime, day or night? Someone who understands what you are going through? If the answer to that question is yes, you are truly blessed.

If you don't have someone you can go to, a pastor, counselor or hospice organization can help you connect with just the right lifeline. Visit *OpentoHope.com* or ████████████ for 24/7 encouragement and support.

Who are your lifelines right now? ■

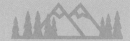

"Admitting there's a problem is an important first step to getting help when you feel discouraged and stuck in grief."

STEP 8

CALLING 911!

Everyone has a unique way of coping with loss. As the world becomes increasingly connected through social media, face-to-face conversations are becoming few and far between. Relying on "likes" and "favorites" won't fill the place in your heart designed for community. If you're feeling disconnected and lonely today, a grief support group can be an excellent place to start.

The most difficult step may be the first one—making the call. Finding the right counselor or support group may take a few visits, but will be well worth the effort. Admitting there's a problem is an important first step to getting help when you feel discouraged and stuck in grief.

What grief support resources are available where you live? Use this space to make a list and keep notes about your experiences with any groups or counselors you visit. ∎

GRIEF SURVIVOR

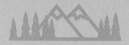

"When people know specifically what you need, they are able to reach out to make your life a little less complicated."

STEP 9

CALL IF YOU NEED ANYTHING

You may have heard the well-intended offer, but chances are you never called back. Here's a straightforward way to communicate exactly what you need.

As you think of something you would appreciate help with, write it on your list. Post it on the fridge.

Your list might include:
- Watching the children for a couple hours
- Raking the leaves
- Technical assistance with the computer
- Driving carpool
- Setting up bills for automatic payment

Whenever something comes to mind, add it to the list. The next time someone asks how to help, snap a photo of the list and send it to them via text or email. If you don't use technology, keep the list closeby so you'll have ideas when someone asks. When people know specifically what you need, they are able to reach out to make your life a little less complicated.

One newly widowed woman shared her list with a church

friend. One day 10 people showed up to clean gutters, move boxes and rake her yard. The entire list was knocked out in an afternoon. What a beautiful reminder that she hadn't been forgotten!

What would go on your list right now? Use these pages to start your list. ■

SURVIVAL TIP

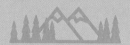

*"One of the healthiest ways
to keep moving forward is to
block off time for mourning."*

STEP 10

TAKE THE DAY OFF

Grief can be hard work and will take time. You may feel like you're working 24/7 to get some relief and healing. One of the healthiest ways to keep moving forward is to block off time for mourning. Clear an entire day on your calendar. Use the day to cry, laugh, write or go for a run—whatever helps you unwind and feel refreshed.

You might want to:

- Go to a quiet place like a lake, beach or mountains.
- Listen to music you love.
- Create something—paint, sing, draw or write.
- Go to a restaurant you and your loved one enjoyed together.
- Take a nap.
- Watch a funny movie.
- Call a friend who always makes you laugh.

Chances are after taking a day for yourself and enjoying a peaceful night, you'll wake up feeling rested and stronger.

Plan your day here. Let your boss, spouse and kids know you're taking the day off. Then take it. ∎

GRIEF SURVIVOR

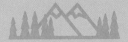

*"Insensitive remarks often
come from people who have
no idea what you're feeling
right now."*

STEP 11

WORDS

At the wake, after the funeral, at the soccer field, you might have heard well-meaning people offer platitudes or explanations to fill the uncomfortable silence. Sometimes there are no words that will make the circumstance better. Sometimes words actually make the situation worse. Maybe you've heard some of these:

Words that don't help

God must have needed another angel in heaven.
You're young. You can marry again.
You can always have more children.
They're in a better place.
You're better now, right?

Insensitive remarks often come from people who have no idea what you're feeling right now. If you're tempted to strike back and set the record straight, it might be wise to take a deep breath and count to ten. Hopefully the well-meaning person will learn from your silence!

Some words that help

I'm so sorry.
I can't imagine how you must be feeling.

I'd love to bring you a meal in a couple weeks.
Please use my beach house if you need it. ■

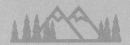

"For some reason, we'll go to the doctor for a broken arm, but we'll try to mend a broken heart with no outside help."

STEP 12

HELP, I'M DROWNING!

Are there days you feel like you're barely hanging on? Feeling overwhelmed can leave us desperate to dull the pain with excessive drinking, eating and busyness. Sadly, when the temporary anesthesia wears off, the pain is still there and usually it's even more intense.

For some reason, we'll go to the doctor for a broken arm, but we'll try to mend a broken heart with no outside help. One of the most courageous steps you can take is admitting you're in over your head. Whether you're experiencing a loss of joy, an inability to concentrate or any other symptom, help is a phone call away. An honest conversation with a healthcare professional or grief counselor is a great next step toward healing.

Additionally, a pastor, priest or rabbi can bring invaluable support and wisdom during a difficult season. Psalm 34:18 is a timeless reminder that you are not alone. "The Lord is close to the brokenhearted. He rescues those whose spirits are crushed."

If you feel like you're hanging by a thread, call someone today. Write about what's going on in your heart on these pages. ■

SURVIVAL TIP

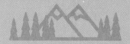

"What if there are stories about your loved one you've never heard?"

STEP 13

THE PERFECT GIFT

What can someone do to make a difference as you begin to heal? You probably have plenty of food, volumes of cards and a house full of flowers, but what kind of gift would genuinely touch your heart?

When you've loved and lost, memories are priceless treasures. What if there are stories about your loved one you've never heard? The next time a trusted friend wants to help, ask them to write a favorite memory and send it to you via mail or email. Can you imagine going to your computer or mailbox and discovering a cherished memory or picture you've never seen before?

As your treasures arrive, put them together in a scrapbook, memory box or journal. You'll be reminded of the difference your loved one made in people's lives.

Who might have a priceless story to share? Make a list on the following pages and begin reaching out to them today. ▪

GRIEF SURVIVOR

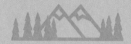

"Revisiting happy memories can be an important step on the path toward healing."

STEP 14

THE MEMORY BOX

The sky's the limit with creating a memory box. Your memory box might be a suitcase, a chest or a storage box. Revisiting happy memories can be an important step on the path toward healing.

You might want to include:
- A fragrance or after shave your loved one enjoyed
- Significant clothing items
- A reminder of a favorite sporting team
- Music
- A journal for writing stories
- A cozy blanket

When children experience loss

Providing a small suitcase for a child can be an excellent way to help them through a difficult season. Having a tangible place a child can go to remember is a great way to start a conversation. Encourage them to draw pictures, save a meaningful video or collect sentimental reminders of the person they're missing. KidGrief.com is an excellent site for kids and their families.

If you create a memory box, what will you include in it?

Write about it here. ■

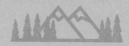

"If grief has taken the wind out of your sails, please know it's OK to not be OK."

STEP 15

IT'S OK TO NOT BE OK

The four-letter word: FINE

During much of life, "fine" may describe your situation accurately. When a casual acquaintance asks how things are going, you may not want to go into a lot of detail. How about when a trusted friend genuinely wants to know how you're coping?

If grief has taken the wind out of your sails, please know it's OK to not be OK. Most of us don't want to feel broken, even temporarily. Keep in mind you are going through one of life's most challenging seasons, and there may be some dark days. Thankfully, the pain will not always be this intense.

Being honest with people who want to help is critical. The next time someone you trust asks how you're doing, tell the truth. Tell them how you're really feeling. Hopefully, today is a terrific day. If not, let someone know.

How are you doing today? Really? You may want to use the following pages to talk about how you're coping. ■

GRIEF SURVIVOR

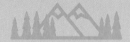

"Writing when life hurts is one of the healthiest ways to begin to heal."

STEP 16

TO WRITE OR NOT TO WRITE?

Not everybody loves to write. For you, writing may feel too much like school. Before you decide you're not a writer, think about this.

Your journal:
- is for your unfiltered thoughts
- will not be graded
- is for your eyes only, if that's how you want it
- doesn't have to be perfect grammar or spelling
- may be stained with tears, and that's OK
- might make you smile or laugh again, and that's terrific
- can be all pictures and no words

Writing when life hurts is one of the healthiest ways to begin to heal. The emotions stuck in your heart now have a way to get out.

You can be completely honest about how you're feeling. Sad? Angry? Relieved? Write about it.

If forgiveness needs to take place, writing is a powerful way to start the process. Maybe you're feeling overwhelmed with thankfulness to have had your loved one in your life. Write about the goodness.

Your journal doesn't have to begin and end here. In a few months or years you may want to add to the story. It's encouraging to read back through your writing and realize the point when your heart began to mend. Use these pages to begin the story. ■

SURVIVAL TIP

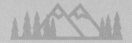

*"When you have a little time
find a cozy place to sit with a
cup of coffee and start to write
about your loved one."*

STEP 17

WHAT IF I FORGET?

The anxiety and stress of sorrow can leave you feeling confused. Hopefully, over time grief-related fog and forgetfulness will lift.

Here are some practical ways to keep your mind and memories clear:

- Say your loved one's name and encourage others to do the same.
- On holidays, tell and retell stories about the person you're missing.
- Look through old photos to stir up memories of vacations and events you may have forgotten about.

Try this:

When you have a little time find a cozy place to sit with a cup of coffee and start to write about your loved one. What did you admire? What made you laugh? Does a particular day or season stand out as fun or memorable? Write every detail you can remember.

Feel free to use these pages to write, draw, save photographs and anything else that helps you remember. ■

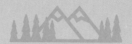

"The best part about hand-prints on your heart is they can never be taken away."

STEP 18

HANDPRINTS ON YOUR HEART

People leave handprints on our hearts. Maybe your loved one's gift of generosity made a lasting impression on you. For some, a hilarious sense humor—and not taking life too seriously is a gift you will always cherish. Or was it their love for animals or children, that you'll never forget?

The best part about handprints on your heart is they can never be taken away. They will forever be part of who you are.

How has your loved one impacted your life and the lives of others? Take your time. Think about the unique and permanent impressions they left on your life.

Write about the handprints left on your heart on the following pages. ■

GRIEF SURVIVOR

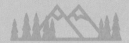

"Taking time to recognize acts of kindness can be a beautiful reminder you are not alone."

STEP 19

GRATITUDE BREAK

After a funeral, it's easy to forget all the ways people step up to offer encouragement. Maybe it was a warm meal or the call that came right when you needed it. Taking time to recognize acts of kindness can be a beautiful reminder you are not alone.

Consider calling or sending a note to someone who has been there for you. Maybe a thoughtful neighbor cut your grass or delivered groceries. Keeping a record of thoughtfulness and expressing thanks is a beautiful way to show gratitude and lighten your outlook on a difficult day. Does someone have a unique ability to make you smile or laugh? Let that person know.

Take a few moments and record the acts of kindness that come to mind on the following pages. ■

GRIEF SURVIVOR

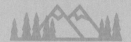

"Grieving 24 hours a day, seven days a week is unsustainable, and will leave you exhausted."

STEP 20

GETTING UNSTUCK

When adversity comes, it's easy to get stuck replaying a mental video of what used to be. Grieving 24 hours a day, seven days a week is unsustainable, and will leave you exhausted.

Even in the midst of intense sorrow, you are probably thankful for something. One of the best ways to redirect your emotions from debilitating worry and sadness to thankfulness and joy is to take time every day to breathe in fresh air. A brilliant sunset or warm breeze can help when you're feeling overwhelmed.

Are there five or ten inspiring people or things in your life? Write about them on the following pages. ■

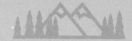

"Every person's path through grief is different, but over time you will see glimmers of light through the darkness."

STEP 21

GLIMMERS OF HOPE

Every person's path through grief is different, but over time you will see glimmers of light through the darkness. Some positive signs may be as simple as going through an entire day with no tears or attending a social function without having a getaway car running in the parking lot.

Anniversaries are good times to reflect and assess how you are doing. If you've been keeping a journal, revisit your earlier writings to see how far you've come.

Some encouraging signs might be:
- smiling and laughing more
- going through the days with fewer tears
- sleeping all night
- feeling more joyful

Noticing steps toward healing, even small steps, can inspire you to continue along the path. Simple things like going for a walk, prioritizing rest and surrounding yourself with uplifting people can help. What step could you take today? ■

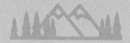

"Rehashing regrets is like riding a stationary bicycle. You go round and round to the point of exhaustion, but don't really get anywhere."

STEP 22

RELEASING REGRETS

Losing a loved one can leave you with a sense of unfinished business. Maybe there's something you wish you could have said or wish you hadn't said.

Rehashing regrets is like riding a stationary bicycle. You go round and round to the point of exhaustion, but don't really get anywhere. If you're feeling frustrated and stuck in regret consider writing about it. An excellent way to clear the air is to write a letter to the person you're missing. Find a time and place you can be alone with your thoughts.

There could be people who need to be forgiven or you could be struggling to forgive yourself for something. Write about it. Forgiveness may not happen overnight and you may have to repeat the process.

Your letter:
- doesn't have to be grammatically correct
- could include some anger
- might make you laugh
- might bring tears
- is for your eyes only (unless you want to share it)

- could be overflowing with gratefulness, or maybe not

You have countless options for releasing your letter when it's complete. You may want to shred it into a thousand pieces, or share with someone you trust. Consider attaching it to balloons and letting it go. One effective way of releasing regrets is to offer them in the form of prayer and ask God to bring peace to your heart and mind.

Use these pages to get started. ■

SURVIVAL TIP

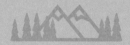

"Thinking ahead can protect you from being caught off guard when a significant day rolls around."

STEP 23

NAVIGATING HOLIDAYS & SPECIAL DAYS

You may have already discovered birthdays, anniversaries and other special days can be particularly challenging after loss. Celebrating holidays the way you always have might feel too painful right now. For the first year or two, you may want to consider changing your traditions as you transition into a new normal.

Thinking ahead can protect you from being caught off guard when a significant day rolls around. Where would you like to spend the day? And with whom? Some families find that reaching out to someone in need is a welcome diversion on an emotional day.

Ideas for navigating special days:
- Buy yourself a gift your loved one might have given you.
- Purchase a gift for someone in need.
- Consider a change of location or menu.
- Listen to music you and your loved one enjoyed together.
- Buy a plant they loved. Plant it somewhere close by.
- Serve at a shelter or soup kitchen.
- Share stories about the person you're missing.
- Take a vacation and come back when the holiday is over.

Is there a special day coming up? Think about what you might do that day. Write about it here. ■

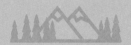

"Helping someone who is hurting can be a stone on the pathway toward healing and can bring meaning to your pain."

STEP 24

TURNING POINTS

As the healing process continues, there will come a day when you hear of a friend who has experienced loss. Whether it's loss of a loved one, a job or even the death of a marriage, losing what's important to us can be devastating.

For months you may not have felt strong enough to offer support for someone else, but now you may feel compelled to reach out in compassion. Helping someone who is hurting can be a stone on the pathway toward healing and can bring meaning to your pain.

As you begin to turn your focus outward, it's good to remember:
- words are not always necessary
- people may not remember what you said, as much as your caring presence in the darkest hours
- spending time with those closest to you is good medicine
- listening to comforting music can help ease weary nerves
- fresh air is great therapy

When you are ready to offer support to someone going through a crisis, what would be a good first step? How could you use what you know now to be a friend to someone in sorrow? ∎

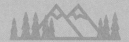

*"Coming up with an original
way to celebrate your loved
one's life can touch others now
and for years to come."*

STEP 25

HEALING BY REMEMBERING

There are countless ways to remember the person you're missing and bring honor to their memory. Is there an organization or church that was a meaningful part of their life?

Consider one of these ideas as a living tribute:
- establishing a scholarship
- coordinating a 5K or 10K walk to raise funds and awareness for a cause or disease research
- donating playground equipment to a local school
- planting a memorial garden with your loved one's favorite flowers
- sponsoring a student on a mission trip in honor of your loved one
- planting a tree or placing a memorial bench in a prominent place

Coming up with an original way to celebrate your loved one's life can touch others now and for years to come. Dream, draw or write about a memorial here. ■

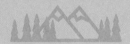

"In an attempt to fill the awk-ward silence we sometimes say crazy things."

STEP 26

LISTEN MORE, TALK LESS

Maybe you're one of the rare individuals who knows exactly what to say in a difficult time of loss. Unfortunately, for the other 99 percent of the world, grief makes us uncomfortable. And in an attempt to fill the awkward silence we sometimes say crazy things. Trying to say something when there are no words to touch the pain can make things worse. When in doubt, listen more. Talk less.

What are the most significant ways you have been comforted? Write about them on the following pages. Take a moment and call or write a quick note to someone who knew exactly how to help. ■

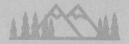

*"A kind embrace will
speak louder than a
thousand empty words."*

STEP 27

COMING FULL CIRCLE

How can you be a friend to someone who is experiencing pain?

Be there.

Even when there are no words to make things better, your presence will speak volumes. A kind embrace will speak louder than a thousand empty words.

Do something.

A person who is hurting may never ask for help. If a thought comes to your mind—whether it's delivering a warm meal—mowing the lawn or providing a gift card, just do it.

Let them talk.

Encouraging conversation about happier times will let the bereaved person know their loved one's life mattered. Consider a blank notebook as a thoughtful, yet inexpensive gift.

Ask for help.

If someone you know is sinking and unable to cope, call for help. A pastor or counseling center is a good place to start.

Use these pages to record ideas for reaching out to someone

during adversity. ■

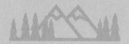

*"What would you like
people to know about your
loved one?"*

STEP 28

TELL THE STORY

What would you like people to know about your loved one? How did their life make a difference to you and others? What are your favorite things about them?

When you have some uninterrupted time alone, sit quietly for a while to collect your thoughts.

You may want to record funny memories you had together. Draw pictures if you'd like to. Save special photos. Take your time and write whatever comes to mind. In a month or two, you might want to revisit the following pages and add to them. ▪

GRIEF SURVIVOR

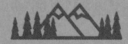

"Each person has their own timeline and unique way of coping with loss."

CONCLUSION

ARE WE THERE YET?

If you took road trips as a child, you probably remember the question parents forever answer: "Are we there yet?" As you regain your equilibrium you may wonder:

How long does grief take?

As long as it takes. Each person has their own timeline and unique way of coping with loss.

Will I always miss my loved one?

Probably so. But, hopefully over time the deep ache will be become more bearable, and memories of the person you're missing will become gentle reminders of the impact they made in your life. Embrace it. It's OK to always miss them.

Why are people rushing me?

People, especially those who have never lost someone close may make insensitive comments about how long your mourning lasts. If someone is in a hurry for you to "be yourself again," remember they did not experience your relationship with the person you're missing. Take as long as you need.

What about closure?

In the words of international grief specialist, Robert Neimeyer, PhD, "closure is for bank accounts, not for love accounts."[2] The purpose of grief is not to "get over it," but to get through the emotions of sorrow, and move toward healing and a full life again. ■

CREDITS

1. Perry Noble, *Overwhelmed*. Tyndale House Publishers, 2014
2. Robert Neimeyer, Ph.D. Dept. of Psychology, University of Memphis

RECOMMENDED RESOURCES

Open to Hope Foundation

Overwhelmed by Perry Noble

The American Widow Project

KidGrief

ABOUT THE AUTHOR

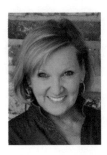

Beth Marshall is wife to Paul and mom to three uniquely awesome grown children — Michael, Caroline and Amy. She adores each of them and their families. In her words, "If we had known how much fun grandkids would be, we would have definitely had them first."

Beth earned a degree in Education from the University of Georgia, then began a two decade career with Delta Airlines. She also served as Pastoral Care Coordinator for NewSpring Church.

The deaths of close family members, and ultimately finding healing and hope through writing led her to write A Time to Heal, a grief journal. Beth is currently a contributing writer for *Open to Hope* and *The Grief Toolbox*; and is honored to serve U.S. military widows as an *American Widow Project* volunteer.

Website: If you found this book helpful, you'll love Beth's website, *www.GriefSurvivor.com*. The site was designed to offer bite sized nuggets of encouragement, connection to world-class resources and a touch of humor to keep it real.

Book Beth to speak: If you are interested in booking Beth for a speaking engagement, please contact *info@GriefSurvivor.com*.